This Book Belongs to

_____

_____

_____

Contact Details

_____

_____

_____

_____

Dedication

This Medication Log Book Journal is dedicated to all the people out there who record their medications and want to document their findings in the process.

You are my inspiration for producing books and I'm honored to be a part of keeping all of your medication notes and records organized.

This journal notebook will help you record your details about your medication.

Thoughtfully put together with these sections to record:

How Are You Feeling Today, Side Effects, How Did You Sleep, I Want To Ask My Doctor, Medication, Dose & much more!

How To Use This Book

The purpose of this book is to keep all of your Medication notes all in one place. It will help keep you organized.

This Medication Log Journal will allow you to accurately document every detail about the medicine you take. It's a great way to chart your course through managing your medication.

Here are examples of the prompts for you to fill in and write about your experience in this book:

1. How Are You Feeling Today? - Write details of how you felt, stress level, any headaches you had, if blood sugar was high, etc.

2. Any Side Effects? - Notes to record any adverse symptoms you had from medication.

3. How Did You Sleep? Diary of monitoring your sleep history, what is helping insomnia, etc.

4. I Am Worried About... Write the things you have concerns about.

5. I Want To Ask My Doctor . . . Record the issues you want to talk to your doctor about.

6. Date & Time Log the time, date & day.

7. Medication Name & Dose - Medicines you take, what time, does it require to be taken with food.

Date: _____

How are you feeling today?

Any side effects?

How did you sleep?

I am worried about...

I want to ask my doctor...

Medication/Dose	Time/ Taken	Time/ Taken	Time/ Taken	Time/ Taken	Time/ Taken	Time/ Taken

Date: _____

How are you feeling today?

Any side effects?

How did you sleep?

I am worried about...

I want to ask my doctor...

Medication/Dose	Time/ Taken	Time/ Taken	Time/ Taken	Time/ Taken	Time/ Taken	Time/ Taken

Date: _____

How are you feeling today?

Any side effects?

How did you sleep?

I am worried about...

I want to ask my doctor...

Medication/Dose	Time/Taken	Time/Taken	Time/Taken	Time/Taken	Time/Taken	Time/Taken

Date: _____

How are you feeling today?

Any side effects?

How did you sleep?

I am worried about...

I want to ask my doctor...

Medication/Dose	Time/ Taken	Time/ Taken	Time/ Taken	Time/ Taken	Time/ Taken	Time/ Taken

Date: _____

How are you feeling today?

Any side effects?

How did you sleep?

I am worried about...

I want to ask my doctor...

Medication/Dose	Time/ Taken	Time/ Taken	Time/ Taken	Time/ Taken	Time/ Taken	Time/ Taken

Date: _____

How are you feeling today?

Any side effects?

How did you sleep?

I am worried about...

I want to ask my doctor...

Medication/Dose	Time/ Taken	Time/ Taken	Time/ Taken	Time/ Taken	Time/ Taken	Time/ Taken

Date: _____

How are you feeling today?

Any side effects?

How did you sleep?

I am worried about...

I want to ask my doctor...

Medication/Dose	Time/ Taken	Time/ Taken	Time/ Taken	Time/ Taken	Time/ Taken	Time/ Taken

Date: _____

How are you feeling today?

Any side effects?

How did you sleep?

I am worried about...

I want to ask my doctor...

Medication/Dose	Time/Taken	Time/Taken	Time/Taken	Time/Taken	Time/Taken	Time/Taken

Date: _____

How are you feeling today?

Any side effects?

How did you sleep?

I am worried about...

I want to ask my doctor...

Medication/Dose	Time/ Taken	Time/ Taken	Time/ Taken	Time/ Taken	Time/ Taken	Time/ Taken

Date: _____

How are you feeling today?

Any side effects?

How did you sleep?

I am worried about...

I want to ask my doctor...

Medication/Dose	Time/Taken	Time/Taken	Time/Taken	Time/Taken	Time/Taken	Time/Taken

Date: _____

How are you feeling today?

Any side effects?

How did you sleep?

I am worried about...

I want to ask my doctor...

Medication/Dose	Time/ Taken	Time/ Taken	Time/ Taken	Time/ Taken	Time/ Taken	Time/ Taken

Date: _____

How are you feeling today?

Any side effects?

How did you sleep?

I am worried about...

I want to ask my doctor...

Medication/Dose	Time/ Taken	Time/ Taken	Time/ Taken	Time/ Taken	Time/ Taken	Time/ Taken

Date: _____

How are you feeling today?

Any side effects?

How did you sleep?

I am worried about...

I want to ask my doctor...

Medication/Dose	Time/ Taken	Time/ Taken	Time/ Taken	Time/ Taken	Time/ Taken	Time/ Taken

Date: _____

How are you feeling today?

Any side effects?

How did you sleep?

I am worried about...

I want to ask my doctor...

Medication/Dose	Time/Taken	Time/Taken	Time/Taken	Time/Taken	Time/Taken	Time/Taken

Date: _____

How are you feeling today?

Any side effects?

How did you sleep?

I am worried about...

I want to ask my doctor...

Medication/Dose	Time/ Taken	Time/ Taken	Time/ Taken	Time/ Taken	Time/ Taken	Time/ Taken

Date: _____

How are you feeling today?

Any side effects?

How did you sleep?

I am worried about...

I want to ask my doctor...

Medication/Dose	Time/ Taken	Time/ Taken	Time/ Taken	Time/ Taken	Time/ Taken	Time/ Taken

Date: _____

How are you feeling today?

Any side effects?

How did you sleep?

I am worried about...

I want to ask my doctor...

Medication/Dose	Time/Taken	Time/Taken	Time/Taken	Time/Taken	Time/Taken	Time/Taken

Date: _____

How are you feeling today?

Any side effects?

How did you sleep?

I am worried about...

I want to ask my doctor...

Medication/Dose	Time/ Taken	Time/ Taken	Time/ Taken	Time/ Taken	Time/ Taken	Time/ Taken

Date: _____

How are you feeling today?

Any side effects?

How did you sleep?

I am worried about...

I want to ask my doctor...

Medication/Dose	Time/Taken	Time/Taken	Time/Taken	Time/Taken	Time/Taken	Time/Taken

Date: _____

How are you feeling today?

Any side effects?

How did you sleep?

I am worried about...

I want to ask my doctor...

Medication/Dose	Time/ Taken	Time/ Taken	Time/ Taken	Time/ Taken	Time/ Taken	Time/ Taken

Date: _____

How are you feeling today?

Any side effects?

How did you sleep?

I am worried about...

I want to ask my doctor...

Medication/Dose	Time/ Taken	Time/ Taken	Time/ Taken	Time/ Taken	Time/ Taken	Time/ Taken

Date: _____

How are you feeling today?

Any side effects?

How did you sleep?

I am worried about...

I want to ask my doctor...

Medication/Dose	Time/Taken	Time/Taken	Time/Taken	Time/Taken	Time/Taken	Time/Taken

Date: _____

How are you feeling today?

Any side effects?

How did you sleep?

I am worried about...

I want to ask my doctor...

Medication/Dose	Time/ Taken	Time/ Taken	Time/ Taken	Time/ Taken	Time/ Taken	Time/ Taken

Date: _____

How are you feeling today?

Any side effects?

How did you sleep?

I am worried about...

I want to ask my doctor...

Medication/Dose	Time/Taken	Time/Taken	Time/Taken	Time/Taken	Time/Taken	Time/Taken

Date: _____

How are you feeling today?

Any side effects?

How did you sleep?

I am worried about...

I want to ask my doctor...

Medication/Dose	Time/ Taken	Time/ Taken	Time/ Taken	Time/ Taken	Time/ Taken	Time/ Taken

Date: _____

How are you feeling today?

Any side effects?

How did you sleep?

I am worried about...

I want to ask my doctor...

Medication/Dose	Time/ Taken	Time/ Taken	Time/ Taken	Time/ Taken	Time/ Taken	Time/ Taken

Date: _____

How are you feeling today?

Any side effects?

How did you sleep?

I am worried about...

I want to ask my doctor...

Medication/Dose	Time/ Taken	Time/ Taken	Time/ Taken	Time/ Taken	Time/ Taken	Time/ Taken

Date: _____

How are you feeling today?

Any side effects?

How did you sleep?

I am worried about...

I want to ask my doctor...

Medication/Dose	Time/ Taken	Time/ Taken	Time/ Taken	Time/ Taken	Time/ Taken	Time/ Taken

Date: _____

How are you feeling today?

Any side effects?

How did you sleep?

I am worried about...

I want to ask my doctor...

Medication/Dose	Time/ Taken	Time/ Taken	Time/ Taken	Time/ Taken	Time/ Taken	Time/ Taken

Date: _____

How are you feeling today?

Any side effects?

How did you sleep?

I am worried about...

I want to ask my doctor...

Medication/Dose	Time/ Taken	Time/ Taken	Time/ Taken	Time/ Taken	Time/ Taken	Time/ Taken

Date: _____

How are you feeling today?

Any side effects?

How did you sleep?

I am worried about...

I want to ask my doctor...

Medication/Dose	Time/ Taken	Time/ Taken	Time/ Taken	Time/ Taken	Time/ Taken	Time/ Taken

Date: _____

How are you feeling today?

Any side effects?

How did you sleep?

I am worried about...

I want to ask my doctor...

Medication/Dose	Time/Taken	Time/Taken	Time/Taken	Time/Taken	Time/Taken	Time/Taken

Date: _____

How are you feeling today?

Any side effects?

How did you sleep?

I am worried about...

I want to ask my doctor...

Medication/Dose	Time/ Taken	Time/ Taken	Time/ Taken	Time/ Taken	Time/ Taken	Time/ Taken

Date: _____

How are you feeling today?

Any side effects?

How did you sleep?

I am worried about...

I want to ask my doctor...

Medication/Dose	Time/Taken	Time/Taken	Time/Taken	Time/Taken	Time/Taken	Time/Taken

Date: _____

How are you feeling today?

Any side effects?

How did you sleep?

I am worried about...

I want to ask my doctor...

Medication/Dose	Time/ Taken	Time/ Taken	Time/ Taken	Time/ Taken	Time/ Taken	Time/ Taken

Date: _____

How are you feeling today?

Any side effects?

How did you sleep?

I am worried about...

I want to ask my doctor...

Medication/Dose	Time/ Taken	Time/ Taken	Time/ Taken	Time/ Taken	Time/ Taken	Time/ Taken

Date: _____

How are you feeling today?

Any side effects?

How did you sleep?

I am worried about...

I want to ask my doctor...

Medication/Dose	Time/Taken	Time/Taken	Time/Taken	Time/Taken	Time/Taken	Time/Taken

Date: _____

How are you feeling today?

Any side effects?

How did you sleep?

I am worried about...

I want to ask my doctor...

Medication/Dose	Time/Taken	Time/Taken	Time/Taken	Time/Taken	Time/Taken	Time/Taken

Date: _____

How are you feeling today?

Any side effects?

How did you sleep?

I am worried about...

I want to ask my doctor...

Medication/Dose	Time/Taken	Time/Taken	Time/Taken	Time/Taken	Time/Taken	Time/Taken

Date: _____

How are you feeling today?

Any side effects?

How did you sleep?

I am worried about...

I want to ask my doctor...

Medication/Dose	Time/ Taken	Time/ Taken	Time/ Taken	Time/ Taken	Time/ Taken	Time/ Taken

Date: _____

How are you feeling today?

Any side effects?

How did you sleep?

I am worried about...

I want to ask my doctor...

Medication/Dose	Time/ Taken	Time/ Taken	Time/ Taken	Time/ Taken	Time/ Taken	Time/ Taken

Date: _____

How are you feeling today?

Any side effects?

How did you sleep?

I am worried about...

I want to ask my doctor...

Medication/Dose	Time/Taken	Time/Taken	Time/Taken	Time/Taken	Time/Taken	Time/Taken

Date: _____

How are you feeling today?

Any side effects?

How did you sleep?

I am worried about...

I want to ask my doctor...

Medication/Dose	Time/ Taken	Time/ Taken	Time/ Taken	Time/ Taken	Time/ Taken	Time/ Taken

Date: _____

How are you feeling today?

Any side effects?

How did you sleep?

I am worried about...

I want to ask my doctor...

Medication/Dose	Time/Taken	Time/Taken	Time/Taken	Time/Taken	Time/Taken	Time/Taken

Date: _____

How are you feeling today?

Any side effects?

How did you sleep?

I am worried about...

I want to ask my doctor...

Medication/Dose	Time/Taken	Time/Taken	Time/Taken	Time/Taken	Time/Taken	Time/Taken

Date: _____

How are you feeling today?

Any side effects?

How did you sleep?

I am worried about...

I want to ask my doctor...

Medication/Dose	Time/Taken	Time/Taken	Time/Taken	Time/Taken	Time/Taken	Time/Taken

Date: _____

How are you feeling today?

Any side effects?

How did you sleep?

I am worried about...

I want to ask my doctor...

Medication/Dose	Time/ Taken	Time/ Taken	Time/ Taken	Time/ Taken	Time/ Taken	Time/ Taken

Date: _____

How are you feeling today?

Any side effects?

How did you sleep?

I am worried about...

I want to ask my doctor...

Medication/Dose	Time/ Taken	Time/ Taken	Time/ Taken	Time/ Taken	Time/ Taken	Time/ Taken

Date: _____

How are you feeling today?

Any side effects?

How did you sleep?

I am worried about...

I want to ask my doctor...

Medication/Dose	Time/Taken	Time/Taken	Time/Taken	Time/Taken	Time/Taken	Time/Taken

Date: _____

How are you feeling today?

Any side effects?

How did you sleep?

I am worried about...

I want to ask my doctor...

Medication/Dose	Time/ Taken	Time/ Taken	Time/ Taken	Time/ Taken	Time/ Taken	Time/ Taken

Date: _____

How are you feeling today?

Any side effects?

How did you sleep?

I am worried about...

I want to ask my doctor...

Medication/Dose	Time/Taken	Time/Taken	Time/Taken	Time/Taken	Time/Taken	Time/Taken

Date: _____

How are you feeling today?

Any side effects?

How did you sleep?

I am worried about...

I want to ask my doctor...

Medication/Dose	Time/Taken	Time/Taken	Time/Taken	Time/Taken	Time/Taken	Time/Taken

Date: _____

How are you feeling today?

Any side effects?

How did you sleep?

I am worried about...

I want to ask my doctor...

Medication/Dose	Time/ Taken	Time/ Taken	Time/ Taken	Time/ Taken	Time/ Taken	Time/ Taken

Date: _____

How are you feeling today?

Any side effects?

How did you sleep?

I am worried about...

I want to ask my doctor...

Medication/Dose	Time/ Taken	Time/ Taken	Time/ Taken	Time/ Taken	Time/ Taken	Time/ Taken

www.ingramcontent.com/pod-product-compliance
Lightning Source LLC
Chambersburg PA
CBHW051030030426
42336CB00015B/2803